From Rejection to Love

The True Story of a Deaf Woman

by

Jennifer A. Hertneky

Dedicated to

Brian Hertneky

My handsome husband who supports me, helps
me, and believes in me and in my writing.
I ask myself every day, "How did I get so lucky
to marry my best friend in the whole world?"

Table of Contents

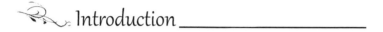

Introduction

I am deaf. I have lived a hard life. At home, I was abused by my family; and at school, I was bullied by other students. My life, mind, and soul were damaged in many ways as a result.

From time to time I have shared my experiences and feelings with friends and, sometimes, even with strangers. My story touched their hearts, and a few of them suggested that I write down my experiences and develop them into a book based on my story. I am so grateful for my friends who have supported me through this difficult project.

One day in the spring of 2014, God called me to write my story and to forgive those in my past who hurt me. My story is only a beginning.

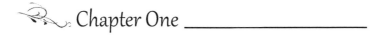 Chapter One _____

My parents were born in Baghdad, Iraq. My family is Assyrian and Chaldean and, therefore, my bloodline Babylonian. My family is Christian.

In the 1980s my dad, Rizkalla, and his twin brother, Paul, fought in the Iraq-Iran War. When the war ended around 1988, my dad made a decision to move from Iraq to Toronto, Ontario, Canada, and make his home there.

In Iraq, my mother, Huda, was raised to work hard, cleaning house, helping her mother, and helping her two brothers and four sisters get ready for school each day. Their poor living conditions required her to not only share one bed with her four sisters, but also to share her clothes, bra, and even her underwear with them. All nine family members managed to live together in their small house of three bedrooms, all sharing the one bathroom.

A dreadfully ugly spirit witch, dark and shadowy, harassed my mother from an early age. The witch would continually call out to my mother, "Huda, Huda." During this time, my mother also suffered from continual strokes that caused her to lose the use of her right arm and, therefore, was prescribed a medication that was supposed to stop the strokes. However, the medication did not seem to work. When she was 14 years old, she quit taking the medication; within a few days, she was back to normal, the strokes having stopped.

My mother fell in love with a guy in Iraq; however, my grandmother did not want my mother to date him.

Meanwhile, my dad's mother called him in 1991 from Iraq to suggest he marry a certain lady in Iraq. He soon made plans to fly back to become engaged to the lady. However, marriage was not to be, as his fiancé broke up with him on the grounds of his continual abuse.

My grandfather, my mom's father, whom I called Baba Jindo met my dad during this time and found out my dad had become a Canadian citizen. He knew it would be beneficial to his entire family if he could get one of his daughters to marry Rizkalla and use him to sponsor his entire family to Canada, running away from Iraq and escaping the suffering and hard life they endured in their war-torn country. So, he made an offer of marriage to one of his three daughters. Rizkalla looked over the three daughters and decided to marry Huda, who later would become my mother.

Huda did not want to marry Rizkalla. She begged her father to not force her into marriage with Rizkalla. However, Baba Jindo explained to Huda that he wanted everyone in his family to move from Iraq to Canada to escape the ravages of war. My parents were married September 28, 1991, in Baghdad.

My mom was soon pregnant with me. She tried to kill me, her unborn daughter, by taking many different kinds of pills during her pregnancy.

While I was still in my mom's womb, I had dreams about what my future would look like. I saw myself as a well-known speaker, giving countless speeches. I saw myself having a beautiful house. I saw angels and had many more dreams that I believe came from God.

I was born on Sunday, December 6, 1992, in Toronto, Ontario, Canada, at Mt. Sinai Hospital. My hair was full and red, and my skin color was white and flecky. None of my family had the same color of hair or skin with which I was born. And, of course, I was also deaf.

I grew up with no love, only hate from my parents. My parents did not accept my being deaf. They did not bother to try to learn how to communicate with me by learning American Sign Language (ASL). In fact, they seemed to actually enjoy abusing me every day for the rest of my life.

I hated my whole self. I didn't love myself because my own family, my parents and siblings, didn't love me. I wished I had never been born on this planet.

It is sad to see many hearing parents who have a deaf child refuse to learn sign language because it is embarrassing or they feel it is shameful to have a deaf child. They give their child no hope that they can have a great future. These children feel neglected and begin to feel rotten from the inside to the outside as though they were cursed from their birth. Deaf people experience such discrimination and oppression every day of their life.

My parents are Christian. They kept showing me movies about Jesus Christ and about loving the Lord and the Father. I hated the Father and Jesus! Every day I wondered if Jesus and the Father really loved me. I hoped they would just let me die.

I was not allowed free speech in my home and among my family. I would be punished, beaten badly, causing deep physical and mental pain and suffering. I was not allowed to go out with my friends, go to my friends' special parties, drive a car, or do anything that "normal" people did.

My two brothers and sister were allowed to do what I wasn't allowed to do because they were hearing, and my parents trusted them to be able to do anything on their own. However, they thought because I was deaf, I was not capable of doing the same things. I was forced to only stay at home and suffer my parents' abuse every day my whole life. I do not have any good memories of my parents or of my siblings.

Every Sunday my family and I attended church at Knox Presbyterian Church in Toronto. I hated church because the people there would speak all the time with no support services for me, such as an ASL interpreter. I couldn't understand at all what they were talking about, so going to church was very boring.

I also hated attending their Sunday School because I couldn't understand most of the time. I never understood what God's Word was. I hated God.

I never got a good grade in Sunday School. I remember my siblings' each passing their test from the class at the church. The teacher from the church gave each of them a certificate, but not to me. A teacher from church explained why I failed Sunday School, which was because I never understood what she taught.

That was the reason why I hated God; I hated the church; and I hated the people there. God didn't reward me. My parents didn't reward me. The people did not reward me. I was a curse.

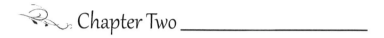 Chapter Two

One day I had a dream that I believe came from God. The dream showed me eating at a table at a large wedding. The table was big and long. I sat there with the rest of my family. My parents, however, lied to everybody about me. That caused the other people to stare at me, looking on me with shame. Of course, my parents had to lie to tell the people how bad I was, further abusing me.

My feelings and emotions were raw, but I had to hold in everything that I felt: the hurt, the pain, the scarring. I wanted to cry. I remember in my dream that I was screaming and shoving the food away onto the floor. It made a mess on the floor and on the table. My cousin was confused at my actions and asked what was wrong. I looked at her and thought to myself that I couldn't stay there any longer.

Another dream I had again involved my parents and siblings treating me hatefully and abusing my feelings. I remember I was innocent of what they were saying about me and crying hard and screaming to the Lord that my family was not the right family for me. I believed God was showing me that I have to leave them for good. I have never had positive dreams about them; they were my nightmare and the destroyer of my life.

*****

My mom's siblings and her father flew to Canada from Jordan. They seemed to be mostly in their 20s. My aunts ran toward me, smiling and with tears in their eyes. My Aunt Mona held me and kissed me a lot. I didn't know her, but I liked the way she kissed me. I felt love from her.

My parents took my aunts, uncle, and Baba Jindo to stay at my Uncle Bashar's apartment. They stayed up all night chatting. However, I went to bed to get some sleep. Aunt Mona came in to check on me and kissed me lightly. I woke up and saw her in the dark in my bedroom. I hugged her. She took me back downstairs, still holding me. Everyone was still up and chatting. They kept it up all night long.

Suddenly, my Uncle Bashar hit my Aunt Mona for no reason other than for fun. I hit Uncle Bashar back. I gave him a mad face. Everyone started laughing. I was so embarrassed and upset. However, at that moment, I started loving my mom's side of the family!

✶✶✶✶✶

One day when I was seven years old, I watched television with the sound on. I did not understand what they were saying on the television, but my parents didn't like closed captions on. I kept watching because I wanted to understand what life was about. It felt as if I was only a robot or a toy without a soul. So, I would just sit down on the floor and watch television every day.

My dad was in the kitchen, and he called me, "Jennifer, Jennifer, JENNIFER!" I couldn't hear him from behind me. Besides, I was focused on the television.

Suddenly, I felt a vibration as though someone was stomping on the floor. Then my dad hit my head so hard, I turned to look at him.

"What did I do?" I cried. "What did I do?"

He hit my face again and again and pulled my long hair. It hurt so badly.

He said, "I called you. You MUST have heard me when I called you. You MUST HEAR ME!" Then he demanded, "Now, say you are sorry to me."

I was sorry for not hearing him. His rule was that I had to apologize to him every time he hit me for not hearing him or for not understanding him. This went on daily.

One day in the spring of 1998, it was warm outside. The sky was blue and sunny. I was watching my siblings ride a bike outside. They smiled, laughed, and enjoyed each other. I ran outside to get my own bike out of the garage. My dad saw me about to ride my bike on the sidewalk. I rode with freedom and happiness as I circled our old house. I enjoyed feeling the wind on my face.

I decided to ride a few blocks away to where my older cousin lived. My dad knew we always rode there and back. I rode my bike a few blocks, and I saw my baby cousin, Sophia, with her grandma. I waved hello to her grandma.

Unexpectedly, my dad drove up in a red car to stop me. I wondered why he needed to stop me.

I was only five houses away from my own house. My dad jumped out of his car and started beating me up. He threw me into the car. I cried from pain and embarrassment. I felt so ashamed. Sophia's grandma saw it happen but didn't want to help by stopping him. That day I learned I would have no love from my extended family.

I ran away two times from my parents' house. I was really tired of my dad's hitting me every day. I was so exhausted. I had many bruises and cuts.

I finally ran to my Aunt Maggie's house. She was my dad's sister. She lived only a few houses away. I told her I needed help. I begged her through my tears, "Please don't ever let me see my dad again. I don't want to go back home. I don't want to see him ever again in my lifetime."

Aunt Maggie calmed me down and wiped away my tears. She said, "Don't worry. I will never let him hurt you." She then went and, without my knowing it, phoned my dad.

I went to Aunt Maggie's family room and started watching television. Suddenly, I saw my dad walk into the family room. I was breathing so hard. He started beating me and grabbed my hair. Aunt

Maggie looked at me, but did nothing, except laugh. My dad thanked Aunt Maggie for calling him, and we left her house, my dad pulling me by the hair. He once again threw me into the car. Once we arrived at home, he continued to beat me more and more.

I chose to stay silent all the time. I knew no one cared about me enough to help me.

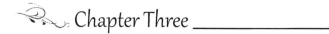 Chapter Three _____

In 1999 I turned eight years old. My cousin, Thamer, picked me up alone every Friday. I don't actually know why he picked me up, but I did enjoy getting away from my dad for an hour.

One day Thamer told my mother she should use red lipstick on my lips. My mother did that. I was very excited to see myself in red lipstick. He drove me around Brampton in his car. As he drove, I noticed he was touching his penis. I didn't understand what he was doing, so I decided to not look at him but, rather, just look out the window. I wondered why he would do that in front of me. He did the same thing again the next time he picked me up.

A few months later, my sister, Lisa, was jumping up and down on my parents' bed. She fell off the bed and hit her forehead on the corner of the bed. It cut her so badly that my parents were unable to stop the bleeding. They took Lisa to the hospital. On the way, my parents dropped off my brothers and me at my Aunt Maggie's house. My cousin, Thamer, was in the house alone.

My brothers and I went to the kitchen and sat down at the table with him. They chatted and laughed; I fake laughed since I could not understand what they were talking about. Thamer asked my brothers if they wanted to go upstairs. They said, "Yes!" He looked at me and asked me if I wanted to go upstairs, too. I nodded my head, "Yes!" I had never been upstairs in Aunt Maggie's house. She never allowed me to go up there, so I was excited and intrigued.

My brothers stood up to go upstairs, but Thamer changed his mind and told my brothers they could not go upstairs. So Thamer and I went upstairs together.

I was curious to see all the bedrooms. Thamer said, "Come to my bedroom," so I went. He closed the door behind me, and I began to feel awkward being alone with him in his bedroom. He took off his pants and showed me his penis. I was very scared as he masturbated in front of me and forced me to touch his penis and masturbate him. I didn't know what to do. He kissed me on my lips and then tried to French kiss me.

It took a while until I stopped him by pushing him backward. I told him I didn't want to do it. He said, "Please."

I told him, "No!" and ran back down the stairs. I was so scared.

A few days later my parents dropped my siblings and me off at his house again. I cried all the way. Once we arrived, I hid from Thamer.

The following day I went to see Aunt Mona's apartment with my mother and siblings. I asked Aunt Mona if she wanted to get married someday. She said, "Yes."

She asked me the same question. I said, "No, I don't want to get married."

My aunt looked shocked and asked, "Why?"

I told her what happened between me and Thamer. I told her not to tell my parents because they would beat me if they found out what happened. Even though she promised she would not tell them, she was very upset and called my mother.

My mother became very upset, too. She told me, "Jennifer, I believe you. Thamer has no right to touch you."

My dad picked us up that night at Aunt Mona's house. My mother had already explained to my dad what happened. My dad looked at me in the back seat of the car, then looked at my mother. "That bitch is a liar. My nephew would never do that to her!"

He then looked at me in the rearview mirror and said, "I don't believe you. Never or ever will I believe you!"

My dad never believed me about anything my whole life. I cried and pounded on the wall. I wished I was strong enough to leave them for good. I didn't have good support at all from anyone. I didn't feel safe being among my family.

*****

I had a couple of important dreams from God. In the first one, I saw myself as a speaker, giving a lot of speeches. I was standing next to the President of the United States. I came to help him. All deaf people were so mad, confused, and frustrated. It was crowded. I wore a business suit.

I remember before I started the speech an angel above me poured a bowl of gold-like water over my head. I felt so calm.

I saw another angel behind me with a light. The angel said, "Go ahead and do the speech. I will help you and support you all the way."

I smiled and signed to the deaf people. I explained to them very clearly. They were so calm and agreed to what I was saying that it stopped the crowd.

In another dream, I was personally having a hard time making friends in Canada. Because I am different like a black sheep, I felt like God was blocking me from having friends. I didn't know why.

I had, again, another dream. I saw myself having a hard time, struggling with the Canadian deaf people I had met. The deaf people said, "If you want to be our friend, then you must go swimming in the water to prove yourself and that you can swim. If you win, we will be friends with you."

I looked at the big pool and deep water. I ran and jumped into the water with my clothes on because I wanted so badly to be friends with them. I am not a good swimmer and can't stay floating in deep water. I swam into the deep water and then started drowning. I blacked out for a long time.

When I woke up, I was shocked to see I was still in the water. I swam to get back up on dry ground. I saw someone whom I had never met grab me and pull me out of the water. I saw it was American deaf people standing in front of me. The Canadian deaf people were standing behind me a far way off. They were looking embarrassed and upset that I made it successfully.

I was confused as to what was going on, so I asked several American deaf people why they were praising me. One of them said, "Don't you remember? Your speeches were very good! You were so good, and you helped save the deaf community!"

*****

One time I told the teachers in public school that I was abused at home and that I didn't feel safe at my house. I was unable to express my true feelings to the teachers because I didn't have access to good communication through having a sign language interpreter. As a result, my teachers didn't believe me. They thought I was just a kid making up lies, that I wasted their time. So, I stayed silent.

One teacher said she was sick of me for not paying attention in the classroom and for not doing my homework. I couldn't understand what the homework was for.

The teachers gave up on me and I was sent to the deaf school in Milton, Ontario, where I was able to communicate in sign language. I was surprised they didn't even give me a suspension for not doing my homework!

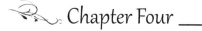 Chapter Four

In the year 2000, I saw a big, beautiful, brown rabbit in the backyard of my old house. It was a male rabbit named Jack. He hopped in my backyard and ate the grass. I stared at him and cried for a long time over my parents' abuse. Finally, I was able to pet the rabbit. I cried a lot because he trusted me to pet him. I felt like he was the only one to believe in me. I continued to pet him and hug him.

My mother came outside into the backyard and said, "Stay away from the rabbit!" She rushed over to me and started beating on me and took me back inside the house. My dad saw Jack outside and yelled at the neighbor across the street to come get his rabbit, so he came and took Jack back.

I cried more and more constantly. I needed that rabbit so badly. He was my best emotional therapy.

One day my dad gave up and took me to the

farm. It was an old farm. An old woman came outside and took us to see her rabbits.

My dad asked me, "Which rabbit do you want?" I was shocked and excited at the same time.

I looked around at the rabbits and felt so badly: too many rabbits in small cages.

"Hurry up!" my dad said.

I hurried and made a choice: a white female named Jenny. I also picked a brown rabbit, Danny, a female, as well.

A few days later my dad took us back to the farm, and I picked another two rabbits. Lisa chose a mixed color female rabbit, and my brother, Edward, chose a black male rabbit, Eddy. Edward also chose two ducks to bring with us back to our home.

At first, we let the rabbits go outside during the daylight, but brought them back into the house when it became dark outside. Finally, my dad made a rabbit hutch in our backyard so the rabbits were able to stay outside all the time. I enjoyed watching them from inside the house and playing with them when I could be outside. Even the neighbor across the street asked my dad to keep Jack because he thought Jack smelled and maybe he would enjoy socializing with the other rabbits. I really did want to have Jack with us, but my dad decided not to keep him.

Over time our collection of rabbits multiplied until we had 40 rabbits at one time. I was happy to have them until my old house was sold in August of 2003, and we moved to a new, bigger house in Brampton, Ontario. My dad gave all our rabbits away. He didn't bother to tell us why; he still refuses to tell me why even today.

*****

My parents were divorced in November of 2003. I didn't even feel sad or upset about it. Actually, I felt happy because I believed they deserved it.

I wanted to live with my mom, not with my dad; but it took a year for my mother to win in court to take me with her.

I hated my dad so much. I believed he was mentally ill, and he was so abusive. The lawyer asked me why I should live with my mom. I tried to explain why, but was unable to fully express myself without an ASL interpreter.

The lawyer only explained to my dad exactly what I had said to him for which he beat me so hard once the lawyer left. I told my dad if he wanted me to stay with him, he needed to stop hitting me. He didn't care about me; he only wanted to keep me living with him.

The rest of my dad's family wanted me to stay with him. I told them I didn't want to live with an abusive dad. Why would my dad hit me in front of them when I said, "No!" I only spoke the truth.

The lawyer seemed to look at me as the lottery: he asked my parents to pay him enough money to win their case to keep me. My dad paid $500. My mom paid $3,500. So, my mom won the case.

*****

I moved to E.C. Drury School for the Deaf in Milton, Ontario, Canada, in September of 2006. I met an amazing teacher, Ms. Bzoney. She was an angel and a life saver. I learned sign language a lot, even though I was older. I felt so comfortable to communicate in that language, but I didn't make any friends until Maryam moved to E.C. Drury School for the Deaf in February, 2007.

Maryam was my first friend at E.C. Drury. She and I chatted a lot. When she was a new student, everybody came to her and made friends with her. I didn't understand why none of them made friends with me when I moved to E.C. Drury. However, I accepted it and moved on.

I wore the same shoes and clothes every day. I tried hard to cover the bruises. No one noticed. I was very thin. My dad was very selfish; he had money but didn't want to spend any on me.

One day Ms. Bzoney could tell there was something wrong. She told my classroom to leave the room. She then looked at me and said, "What's wrong with you?"

I felt something must be up, and it scared me, so I simply said, "Nothing."

She said, "Try me."

I said, "I will be wasting my breath on you—no one will believe me."

She said, "I believe you."

I told her what happened at home with my family. She listened from the beginning to the end. I couldn't even stand to look at her. I looked down and just knew she would say, "I don't believe you."

Instead, she said, "Follow your heart! Don't let them control you. It is your body, not theirs."

I had thought wrong. It was the first time in my life that I discovered I had a heart and a soul! I started crying and hugged her hard. I told her, "Thank you for believing me!"

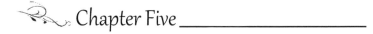 Chapter Five _____

In November, 2006, I finally got out of my dad's house and started living with my mom, Baba Jindo, and my mom's siblings. I made a promise to myself that I would never see my dad ever again. All I wanted was to be free and find happiness.

I was finally living with my mom and enjoying the time I spent with my aunts, my uncles, and Baba Jindo. We made many good memories. They took me out to eat a lot. They helped me to know that my uncles and aunts cared for me.

My mom met a new boyfriend at her work. She hung out with him a lot. After two years my mom took me away from her siblings and her father. She still wouldn't let me go out with my friends, have or drive a car, or go to parties, forcing me to stay home all the time.

On my fifteenth birthday, my mom and her boyfriend bought me a Maltese puppy. Her name was Maggie. Maggie was a beautiful baby girl. She helped me to "hear" when someone was at the door knocking. We slept together every night.

*****

In the ninth grade of high school, I joined a soccer team to play in the Deaf Soccer Tournament, competing with other deaf schools in Canada and the USA. I realized I needed a passport in order to go to Rochester, New York, to participate in the tournament. Since I was under 18 years old, the passport application required my dad's signature. I got upset that I didn't even have a choice, but my mom took me to see him in person. I wondered why I had to see him all over again.

My dad was happy to see me. My siblings were also happy to see me. They missed our mom.

I hated to see my dad's ugly face again. He looked the same. He looked as if he was full of demons. His house smelled really bad, and he was a hoarder of wood in his living room, basement, and office.

I explained to him why I needed to have a passport to go to the USA. My dad refused. I fought with him. My siblings were shocked to see me get into a fight. My brother, Daniel, finally stepped in and fought my dad for me.

My dad finally gave in and agreed for me to get a passport. Of course, my dad always listened to my hearing siblings more than he listened to me.

I asked my dad to give me my birth certificate. He said he would give it to me at school the next morning. My siblings then ran to see my mom and chatted with her.

The next day a teacher called me out of swimming class to see my dad. I looked upset as I walked with the teacher to see him. She stopped me and said, "I know that look. I don't know you, and you are not one of my students, but I hate my dad, too."

She explained to me about her terrible experience with her father. She understood how I felt by the look on my face. I looked at the floor, thinking, then looked back at her. "Please don't believe every word my dad says!"

She agreed and said, "I will be on your side."

We went to see my dad with a sign language interpreter. My dad gave her a copy of my birth certificate. She made a face and said, "No, I need a real birth certificate." She went on to explain to my dad that it was the law to have an original birth certificate to go through the border.

My dad gave her the original birth certificate. I looked at the deaf teacher and said, "Thank you." I then went back to swim class.

*****

I hated the deaf school. The deaf students there bullied me every day because of where my family was from, Iraq. Also, I'm hard of hearing, not profoundly deaf like they were; my signing skills didn't meet their standards. There were many other reasons, as well.

I cried in my bed every night before I went to sleep until I graduated from high school. I ate my sandwich from my lunchbox in the lobby, not in the café, because I didn't feel safe to go in there for their bullying. It was so hard for me to find good friends there. I had a few good friends, but they always left me out. I lost some friends because others caused us to have a problem, making us not to be friends anymore.

I had a crush on a guy at E.C. Drury for quite a long time. One day my friend dared me to say "I love you" in sign language to him. I was very shy, so at first, I didn't want to do it. Finally, I did. Later, I told him it was just a joke, and he told me he knew I was joking the whole time. I smiled and asked him out for a date. He turned down my invitation, saying he was not interested in me. He went on to say that besides not being interested in me, he worried about what others would think if we got together, and it would make him look bad. I felt sad and hopeless.

A few weeks later I was struggling and feeling frustrated with my science homework as I worked on it in the lobby. I happened to see him chatting with some friends. Even though I was shy, I made a decision to be brave and ask him to help me finish my homework. He agreed to help me, but then his friends began to mock him, saying, "Why don't you date Jennifer?" Suddenly, he stopped helping me and said, "No way!"

I was speechless. I thought to myself, "I wish I was beautiful."

*****

One night I had another dream from God. I was driving a dark gray SUV. I parked at a big house and hopped out of the car. I grabbed a little girl that looked to be about three years old. She had long, curly hair; she looked so beautiful. She smiled and laughed. I remember in my dream, however, that I looked sad.

The little girl and I went inside the big house. I took her to the bathroom and put her in the tub. The bathroom looked so very nice. I washed the little girl's whole body. After her bath, I covered her with a white towel. She looked at me and smiled. She said, "I love you, Mama." I woke up suddenly, feeling shocked. For a moment, I thought it was real.

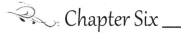 Chapter Six _____

I wanted to be a massage therapist. I went to my principal, Tony, and asked him to please allow me to take a chemistry class so I could be a massage therapist in the future. Tony thought I couldn't do it because of my English. I was sad and went to the library to study and work on my homework on my own.

The librarian came to me and asked, "What's the matter?"

I explained to her about what happened with Tony. She looked at me and told me she believed in me and that I could do it, that I had a future. I told her I felt like I had no future.

She went to Tony to fight for me. Finally, Tony accepted the idea and sent me to a hearing class for science with an ASL interpreter. I was excited and thanked her for her help. I promised her I would not fail her.

I went to the hearing science class every day, and I learned it was much harder than I expected it to be. There was a big difference from the deaf school. In deaf classes, students are not taught at a hard level, so this class was a challenge for me. I enjoyed it a lot.

However, at the end of the semester, I failed the librarian. I look at my past and wish I could have had a lot of help and support so I would not have failed.

I graduated as a senior in E.C. Drury at the end of June, 2012. I headed to George Brown College (GBC) the following January to study makeup artistry. I actually had no idea what my future looked like.

*****

I had a dream from God. The background looked like Heaven. I saw bright white everywhere. I saw a tall man with brown hair and white skin, wearing a white suit. He had huge wings; the wings were so beautiful. I couldn't see his face; it seemed blurred.

He came to me. He signed and sang, "Would you dance, dance with me?"

He grabbed my hands and pulled me to get closer to him. I pushed him away because I was carrying my pain from the past. I looked so sad. I walked away and then stopped. I could feel the vibrations from the music. So, I turned back to look at him.

"Come, dance with me," he sang.

"Today is my last day in the world," I cried.

He grabbed my hands and we danced together. I cried so hard, looking at him. He took my pain away. I felt Heaven was singing. The light was shining so brightly that I had to close my eyes.

*****

During my first year at GBC, I went to the Deaf Club in Toronto for the first time. I remember I wore 1970s-style clothes. It was my very first time to be in a club and see people dancing and drinking. I was very excited to be able to meet new people. I could feel myself smiling big.

A hearing guy who was tall with brown hair and a light tan stared at me. I made a face back at him.

I found it weird, but I was chatting with new deaf people. I saw a handsome guy with dirty blond hair and blue eyes, wearing a nice hat. He had a nice beard and a beautiful smile. He accidentally hit me and said he was sorry. I smiled at him and said it was okay. I felt very shy at the moment and thought about how much I really liked his smile. I couldn't stop staring at him while I was chatting with my friends.

We left the dance floor and went over to the bar. My friends bought me a drink. I tried to act like a party girl and thought I was smart by drinking. I chose to pretend to be worldly, but that is not the real me.

The guy I had seen didn't come over to me or try to talk to me. I waited, hoping he would come over. So finally, I went to him.

He told me his name was C.J. I told him my name and asked him where he was from because I had never seen him around Toronto. He explained he had come to Toronto from Alberta, Canada, for his art show. He said that he worked with welding as art.

We chatted for quite a long time. I noticed a hearing man kept looking at me. I suggested to C.J. that we move to another spot because the man kept looking at me, so we moved. The hearing man looked really angry, and he walked up and pushed C.J. backward. C.J. pushed him back.

I grabbed C.J.'s shoulder and said, "Please, don't fight!" However, they got into a fight inside the club. I was scared and shocked; it was the first time I had seen an actual fight. Then I thought, "Oh, my gosh! Does C.J. like me?" The guys were fighting over me!

My friends stopped the fight. I looked at C.J., feeling so in love. I grabbed his arm and pulled him toward me. "Are you okay?" I asked.

He said, "I'm fine."

He told me he could see light in my heart. Instinctively, I covered my heart with both of my hands; I was shocked that he could see something. I asked him if he was spiritual. He said he was.

At that moment I felt like maybe he was the one for me. I was so young, and I felt so in love too fast; but I thought he was the one. We talked all night long. Finally, I told him I had to go home. He asked me to add him as a friend on my Facebook page, which I did.

I went back home to Brampton from Toronto at 7 a.m. I believed I would be successful in having him in my life. I felt such joy and happiness. We talked on the phone every day for three months.

I decided to go see him for his birthday in June and stay a week. I paid for the flight and flew to Calgary, Alberta, from Toronto. I was very excited but ended up being very sad in the end.

After getting to know me, he didn't love me anymore. He didn't seem to be the same person who used to talk to me. I cried at his house every day. I didn't laugh at his jokes. I kept thinking I needed to stay positive; he would like me again later.

I felt so awful, wishing I was the best lady for him. I wished I was the perfect answer for his needs. I failed. I failed. I failed to win him over.

The last night we had together he told me that if we were to get back together, I needed to travel, meet older people, and find happiness.

I returned to my home in Brampton from Alberta. I was happy to be at home, but I missed him. I tried to talk to him like we talked on Facebook before, but he stopped talking to me. I carried so much sadness around inside me. I knew he would never talk to me again for the rest of my life.

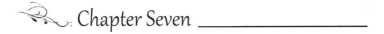 Chapter Seven _____

I decided to go to New York City to meet new deaf people at the Deaf Expo. I met a few guys from the Middle East. They led me to some of their friends. I saw a tall, handsome man with curly black hair and a beautiful smile. His name was David.

I was to meet a friend at the food court, so I hurried to get there. David was also at the food court; I found it odd. We chatted together. He asked if I would hang out with him the next day before I returned to Canada. I smiled and said, "Sure." I was hoping he would like me. I tried to be perfect.

The next day David and his best friend, David B, picked me up at my friend's house where I had slept over. I was very excited to hang out with new friends. They showed me around New York City. I had so much fun with them all day, and we went to many different areas around the city.

That night at the subway, David said, "I like you."

I said, "I like you, too."

He smiled and kissed me. I looked at him and felt so in love. I hoped he would not hurt my heart like C.J. had done.

I returned back home in Canada. I missed David. We texted on the phone every day. I decided to surprise him with a visit to New York City. I went to his house in November, 2013. I stayed with him for three days. We went out to the bar, and he showed me his college. After the three days, he asked me if I would stay in a relationship with him even if he was an alcoholic. I said, "Yes, I will always love you, no matter if it is good or bad." He looked at me but remained silent.

I asked him, "What's wrong?"

He said, "Nothing." Then we hugged.

I went back home from New York City. I tried to text him as I wanted to stay in touch with him. However, he stopped talking to me. It hurt me more and more.

*****

I first met Melissa J. at GBC. She came from Jamaica. She had brown skin; short, wavy black hair; and brown eyes. She came to GBC to study to reach her dream. I met her at a friend's birthday party at the club where we used a hookah together.

We didn't see each other again until I went back to GBC. We became close friends after we talked about someone we both didn't like at the computer lab in the basement.

Melissa J. helped me a lot through the years—through good and bad. We never fought. She loved me for who I was. She witnessed to me every single time I went through all the problems and situations with my family, my roommate, and more. She even stood up for me when some guys came up to bully me.

We went out to eat at many different restaurants to which we had never before been, curious to taste the different foods of various cultures. Toronto is very diversified, full of many immigrants from all over the world who brought their cultures with them. It feels like a second home to those from many different countries. That is why it was so much fun to adventure around Toronto, downtown, uptown, and even the surrounding cities.

Melissa J. was there for my birthday on December 6, 2015, at Dave and Buster's. She even surprised me with Pakir on my birthday a year later in Wasaga Beach. I had so much fun with her. I was lucky to have Melissa J. as she is the only one who stayed close to me and talked to me daily. She was like a sister to me.

*****

I had a hard time looking for a job because of the communication barrier, being that I was deaf. Hearing people who never experience the deaf culture may think deaf people don't deserve to get a job. However, when we don't have a job, we are poor. Hearing people who have a job find it easier to get money. I found it so unfair.

I finally went to Deaf Services and asked a deaf worker named David for help. He helped me fix my resume. A few weeks later he helped me apply for a job at Target. It worked! I got my first job at Target on November 28, 2014, in Brampton for seasonal holiday work.

I enjoyed working with Ida, a deaf lady I knew

from my old neighborhood. She lived only a few blocks away from my dad's house.

My manager at Target told me I could continue working there after the holiday season. I was excited! I thought it was a great experience for me. However, an Indian woman on my team didn't like to work with me just because I was deaf. I never bothered her, but she said I did. She mocked me. I felt sad because no one at work stood up for me. Six months later I was sad to see Target shut down in Canada.

Later I worked as a waitress for a wedding in Mississauga, Ontario, and I also worked for a while at a five-star hotel. I enjoyed getting to know how the real world looked.

*****

I was fighting so hard with my mom every day, and I was getting tired of her not letting me get a driver's license. I tried to express my feelings to her. She refused to listen to me. She allowed my siblings to drive a car but believed I could not drive because I was deaf. She would pick up and drop off my siblings from their work, but she would never pick me up or drop me off anywhere. She would say I could take the bus.

One late night in February, there was no bus. I called my mom to come pick me up. She couldn't have cared less. It was so cold and snowing heavily. The ground was covered in ice. I only had a thin jacket. I walked for an hour and a half to get home.

On another day I called my mom around 1:30 a.m. to pick me up in Mississauga because there was no bus running that late. She refused. I cried at the cold. I didn't have any money on me.

I called my friend, Kevin, to see if he could pick me up. He didn't answer his phone. So, I texted him, "I will kiss you if you will pick me up." He answered he would come pick me up. I stood at the bus stop, waiting for Kevin for 20 minutes. He finally arrived and drove me home. We were so quiet in the car. When he stopped at my house, I thanked him and kissed him on the cheek. He later texted me that he thought I would kiss him on his lips. I knew he would say that.

I am a victim of my life. My mom never makes me happy. My parents are not good role models for me.

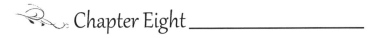

Chapter Eight

On my 21st birthday, it was my first time to host my birthday party and have friends meet me at Dave and Buster's. My friend, Long, picked me up and gave me a present. It felt so good to receive a present. My parents never gave me presents on my birthday or at Christmas. I felt so special, and it put a smile on my face.

I put Long's present on my bed in my bedroom, and I left to go to Dave and Buster's. I enjoyed the time so much. After the party, Long dropped me off at my house. It was snowing and very cold. I ran inside to get warm.

I saw my mom, Lisa, and Daniel in the family room. I ran upstairs to my bedroom and found the present, opened, on the bed. It hurt me so much; it was not okay for someone to open my present! It was my birthday! I was so frustrated and angry! I ran downstairs and told my mom.

"Mom, did you see Lisa open my present? It is my birthday! I am supposed to open it, not Lisa!"

My mom gave me a bad look.

I said to my mom, "Why are you always blaming me all the time? Why do you keep looking down at me all the time? Why do you allow Lisa to touch my stuff and I cannot? You told me if something happens, I should tell you. So, I did. Now, you give me that ugly face. This communication is such a barrier to me."

Daniel said, "Stop talking!"

I looked at Daniel and said, "I am only expressing how I feel."

My mom answered, "No, you are not allowed to express how you feel."

I realized then that no one in my family cared about me. They allowed my siblings to express their feelings, but I was not.

Daniel then hit me. I hit him back and yelled for him to stop. I threw my present at the wall and looked at Lisa.

I was so tired of their blaming me. When something bad happened to them, they used it against me. They didn't care if I was innocent. They always wanted to hurt me and hurt my feelings, which made them happy.

Lisa gave me her pure devil face. I said, "You won. Are you happy?"

I continued to throw things at the wall. Daniel hit me again. I had really bad bruises on my arms and legs from him.

My mom and Lisa laughed so hard. I had had enough! I ran outside. It was very cold. I tried to find the police station, but it was too cold. I didn't make it to the police station.

Daniel came outside and searched for me. When he found me, he beat me so badly that I blacked out. I woke up in my bedroom and cried.

I texted my two best friends for help. My friends called the police to come help me. Two policemen came. I told them I needed an ASL interpreter. I knew there was no other way for me to communicate with them.

My mom talked to the police as if nothing had happened. They did not bother to listen to my side of the story, and they took me to the hospital without explanation. I found out later they had taken me to a mental hospital. Lack of communication!

I couldn't believe I was actually in a mental hospital. They ignored my pain and suffering. I wanted to report Daniel's abuse, but they simply took me to a mental hospital, thinking I was mentally ill. The hospital refused to get me an ASL interpreter to make it possible for me to clearly communicate with them. They ignored my pain and suffering, as well. I fought with them all day long.

A black woman who worked at the hospital told me she was a counselor. I told her, "Sure, you are a counselor. Get me an ASL interpreter." My mom had told them I didn't need an ASL interpreter because I could talk, so the black lady had an attitude with me.

I wondered why I bothered. No one was willing to listen to how I felt. The police and the hospital made a choice to listen to my mom's side of the story and to her lies because it was easier for them to believe her rather than to try to communicate with me.

Later, I made a report to the police department and filed a complaint with the hospital. Canada's system for deaf access to an interpreter and for deaf rights are very bad. They do not have the Americans with Disabilities Act (ADA) as America has. Canada needs a similar law to have DEAF RIGHTS laws to protect deaf individuals from police, government public offices, and all kinds of businesses. Once Canada has such a law, the deaf can have improved access to all the resources needed to allow deaf individuals to feel more equal with the rest of the people in Canada.

*****

In April of 2015, I decided to move out of my mom's toxic house. I did so late at night. I decided to live with an old deaf man as a roommate. His name was Marco. He lived in Toronto.

It was a huge mistake for me to live with Marco. He lived in a very old house. It smelled like fish mixed with mold. There was too much dust in his house. The backyard was small and muddy. It was a really horrible experience.

I lived there for three months, sleeping in a bedroom in the basement. I searched for a job and hung out with my best friend, Melissa J. She lived only a few blocks away.

Marco harassed me to have sex and to shower with him every day. I kept saying, "No." He bothered me again and again. I tried to avoid him. I became scared of him.

One day Marco told me he paid $1,000 to have sex with a deaf lady. I found it gross and scary. Marco said he was willing to pay me $10,000 if I would be willing to have sex with him. I denied his offer. He was very angry.

A few days later I accidentally found many pictures of deaf, naked women in his bedroom. The naked pictures were lying right there on a table just inside his bedroom. I looked for more pictures, curious as to who these women were. I did not feel comfortable.

I felt awful when I discovered a picture of a deaf, naked teenager. I knew the girl, so I texted her and told her she was underage and should make a report to the police. She didn't want to report him to the police; she wanted to remain his friend. There was nothing more I could do to help her. She made the wrong choice for allowing him to see her body.

I remember he told me he watched underage porn often. He forced me to watch porn even when I refused. I continued to refuse to watch porn because it was very gross to me to see the people on there naked. Marco wanted me to have an open mind and said it was okay for us to talk about dirty stuff, but I continued to refuse him. He became angry with me because I would not sleep with him in his bedroom.

After three months of being Marco's roommate, I left. It felt so good leaving his horrible house. Marco threatened that I would fail, that I would never get married, and that my money would be cut. I only nodded at him. Melissa J. came to pick me up. Marco wanted me to stay, but I didn't want to stay there with him because he was a toxic, very sick man.

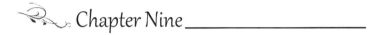 Chapter Nine

In September, 2015, I moved to Wasaga Beach, Ontario to be a roommate with Tasha, whom I had known since my childhood at Great Lakes Public School in Brampton. We grew up together and we played "It" a lot with the hard-of-hearing kids. I had not seen her for six years when I moved to the deaf school and she stayed behind at the hearing school. I had found her on Facebook after six years of separation.

Tasha was tall and had blue eyes and white skin. She was hard of hearing, so she could hear some. She was able to talk very well.

Tasha's mom was awesome! She raised Tasha very well, spoiled her, and loved her as she was. Tasha had two beautiful daughters when I moved in and later had a handsome son. She had a lot of cats in her house. I always kissed the cats and made them scared of me. I wished I could have been Tasha's roommate much earlier.

Wasaga Beach is so beautiful. Tasha and I loved walking around and eating at Tim Horton's, a famous coffee shop in Canada. We chatted every night after her daughters went to bed. We even got to go to Canada's first bar, The Ranch, in Barrie, Ontario, where we enjoyed drinking and line dancing with our friends.

I had many good memories with Tasha. She knew me well and trusted me.

*****

Graham was an ex-boyfriend whom I dated for only about two weeks way back in the ninth grade. He contacted me and asked me if I would go with him to a house party in Rochester, New York. It was my first time to actually go to a house party. I was nervous and scared, but I went ahead to give it a try.

When we first arrived at the party, I saw a girl, another Melissa, whom I did not personally know. I only knew her from something that happened back in 2007. I had just gotten my first MSN account. I tried to think of a nickname for my account. I input "Juicy Jexy Homeworld." Three seconds later I decided I didn't like it, so I changed it to "Jexy Homeworld." I saw that a girl added me on MSN late that night. It was the girl, Melissa, who was at the party. She messaged me.

"Hello. Who is this?" I asked.

"You copied my nickname," Melissa said.

"I didn't copy your nickname. How did I copy your nickname?" She seemed creepy and quite bossy. She didn't answer. So, I messaged, "Why would you add me and immediately try to start a fight with me about your nickname?"

She answered, "Alex told me." Alex was a deaf Mexican boy whom we both knew.

I ended up blocking her. I found it so immature and annoying.

As soon as Melissa saw me at the party, she started texting someone. I got bad vibes from her. I walked to another room and texted Michael and asked him to come to the party because I was bored. Michael replied that he was on his way.

When Michael arrived, he started searching for me in the large crowd. I saw him and waved at him. He came over to me and we chatted for about half an hour.

I noticed four Canadian girls arrive. I didn't realize they were looking for me; they brushed past me. However, Melissa saw me and pointed me out to the girls. They tried to argue with me in front of everyone, but I stood silent. They were upset because I had added Rami, an Iraqi guy, as well as several other Iraqi guys as friends on my Facebook page.

When I added Rami to my Facebook, he had happened to see my video with sign language I had posted on Facebook. He inboxed me and said, "My girlfriend is deaf and knows sign language."

I was shocked as it was my first time to hear of an Iraqi guy dating a deaf woman. "Do you know sign language?" I asked curiously.

"No," he answered.

A few weeks later I saw Rami's girlfriend, Nay, at a restaurant in Toronto. She came to me and asked if I had added Rami to my Facebook. I was curious why she would come up to me like that. She looked me up and down as if I was nothing. Later, I texted Rami that I was not happy how he told her about me and to not ever do that again. He apologized and went on to tell me how bad a person Nay was. I accepted his apology.

I asked the girls trying to pick a fight with me at the party, "Do you feel better now by trying to fight with me in front of everyone?"

"I broke up with him because of you," Nay said. "I already have proof of your conversation to my girls. You hate deaf people." She continued, "Why are you here? You won't find love because no one at this party likes you."

She thought I hated deaf people? I actually hate how deaf people make drama.

Four weeks later Rami tagged me and Nay on Instagram. I was not able to check my phone until three hours later. The tag was gone. I inboxed Rami and asked him what the tag was about. He said, "Thank God you didn't see the awful messages Nay and the girls wrote about you." Rami found no reason to hurt me, so he had removed the messages. It upset him, and he apologized to me again.

I said to Rami, "I don't understand what their problem is."

He said he didn't understand, either.

I asked him, "Is it true she broke up with you because of me?"

He said, "No, that is not true. None of this is your fault. Nay doesn't make any sense."

I agreed. However, at that moment, I decided to block him on Facebook for Nay's sake.

I remember thinking how I wished my best friend, Melissa J., was there to see how awful the girls were acting. I didn't have any close friends there.

The party was crowded with deaf people partying hard, smoking weed, fighting, and playing games. I realized partying hard wasn't for me.

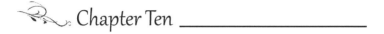 Chapter Ten _____

Somehow God guided me to go to the Rochester Institute of Technology (RIT) in Rochester, New York. It was there that I would meet the man who would become the love of my life. I did not have any experience of having a long-term boyfriend; I always wanted one so badly. I wanted to get married and have a baby.

I made some new friends at RIT in the gym when I went to watch a basketball game. I saw many handsome men there. Then I saw a handsome man with brown hair, white skin, and brown eyes. It was Brian Hertneky, chatting with another man named Joseph.

At that moment I felt the Holy Spirit pushing me to meet him. I felt butterflies in my stomach, but I couldn't stop staring at him. I walked around in the lobby. I felt it again: like the Holy Spirit pushing me and making me turn to look at him.

Finally, Brian stopped chatting with Joseph and walked toward his friends in the gym. I was scared and thought, "What if he is not interested in me? What if he already has a crush?" I kept worrying about what was going to happen, afraid something bad would happen.

I finally stopped thinking and went toward him. I patted him on his shoulder. He turned his head around to look at me. I told him my name and that I was a fan of his. I don't know what I was thinking! I talked so weird and felt so awkward. I turned to walk back to the lobby. Then I turned around to check on him; he was smiling.

The next night there was a big party. I walked around the gym and I accidentally hit a big guy's shoulder. I said I was sorry, but he made a face at me and had a bad attitude.

"Why are you looking at me like that?" I asked defiantly.

I walked toward some ladies at a booth taking pictures. A guy named Samir caught up with me and asked if I was from Iraq. I was shocked and answered, "Yes."

He looked so excited. He said, "I found a guy for you. He's from Egypt." He led me to him and introduced him as Michael. Samir told Michael, "I found an Iraqi, and you should marry her! She is beautiful!"

I took one look at Michael and ran off. I thought it was the same guy who had made a face at me, but it was not; it was a misunderstanding.

Michael ran up to me and started walking beside me. He tried to tell me he was not the guy who had made a face at me. I ignored him and continued to walk to the basement, but he was very persistent to get my attention. Finally, I gave up and looked at Michael, wondering if he was the one.

We chatted a little to get to know each other. Michael took me to his two best friends on the dance floor. I had no interest in watching others dance, so I said, "I'm going back downstairs to play pool with the guys."

Michael agreed to let me go, but he stopped me again and asked for my phone number. That was the first time anyone had asked for my phone number. I thought, "Is he actually asking for my number? Does he like me?" I looked as serious as I could as I gave him my number.

I then went back downstairs to play pool. I saw Brian near the bar. Again, the butterflies came to my stomach. I felt the Holy Spirit pushing me and saying, "He is the one."

I stopped playing pool and told my friend, Thomas, "Give me a minute. I will be back, I promise."

I walked toward Brian and asked him if we could have our picture taken together. I was surprised when he said, "Yes." I gave my friend, Lance, my phone to take the picture. After the picture, Lance said to Brian, "You are famous!" I smiled and ran back to play pool.

Some deaf people saw what happened and laughed. Brian said, "Stop it," but he laughed, as well.

He wondered who the girl was; why had she come to him? Why did she seem so shy? He wished he would have had a chance to chat with her and get to know her. He wondered if he would ever see her again.

The next day Brian went to a bash party. He chatted with two friends, talking about how to make a better blog. Then he told them about a girl he had met named Jennifer. He said he had just happened to see her and that she was shy, but smiled at him.

She had asked for a picture of them together and Brian had agreed. After they took the picture, she had thanked him and then walked away. Brian explained to his friends that he never had a chance to talk to her, but he had been thinking about her ever since.

Finally, I left Rochester. I took a Greyhound bus to go back home to Toronto. I received a text from Michael asking how I was feeling. I was excited to hear from him, so I answered him right back. I was hoping he was the one for me.

He said he was curious and wondered if we got married, would I go to church with him. I answered him, "No." He was shocked.

He asked if I would be willing to go to church with our kids. I said, "The kids can go with you, and I can stay at home." He said then he was not interested in me. I was disappointed and upset, wondering why I couldn't find the love of my life.

I arrived home from the long trip. I screamed and cried. I yelled to Jesus and asked Him why He always blocked my path. I wanted to have a family so badly. I didn't want to live with my family forever. I was so tired. I gave up my heart and my soul to Him, Jesus. I was on my knees, begging Him to show me the love of my life.

I went to take a shower. After the shower, I fell to the floor, crying. Then I felt God take away my pain, and at that moment I knew the Father would bring to me the love of my life.

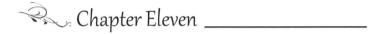 Chapter Eleven _____

Brian, whom I had met earlier at RIT in Rochester, New York, returned to his home in the USA. For the next several months he traveled around the States. When he finally got back home, he got on his computer at his office. He checked Facebook and happened to see my picture as a mutual friend of another friend of his. He sent a friend request to me.

I was still in Toronto. I checked my phone and saw that Brian had sent me a friend request on Facebook, which I accepted.

It was three months before we ever talked, but we finally started chatting by webcam to get to know each other better.

Brian took me to Disney World in Florida in April, 2016, for the first time. Hervin, a very good friend of Brian's, came along with us. I had so much fun in Florida. I was away from my problems and felt peace of mind and happiness.

Brian proposed to me in front of Hervin while we were in Florida. I said, "Yes!" In July I found out I was pregnant, and September 8, 2016, we were married at the deaf church by a deaf pastor, John Graham. On September 26 we had a big, beautiful wedding. Everyone loved the Iraqi foods we served.

At the same time, I was having many problems with my parents, who were trying to control me and my relationship with Brian. When I was two months pregnant, we had a big fight that lasted two days. I began vomiting blood. My mom refused to take me to the hospital.

Brian was in Pennsylvania at the time. I finally gave up trying to get my mom to take me to the hospital and called Brian. I asked him to call the hospital for me. Brian called 911 to get an ambulance to me at my mom's house to take me to the hospital. I was at the hospital for four hours.

Canadian hospital service is very slow, but I was finally able to see the doctor. He said I almost lost the baby and I could have died, as well. The doctor said I was very lucky and that I must stop the fighting at home. I didn't want to fight with my parents, but they were always trying to control everything I did and they seemed to love to fight with me. I had no support.

My beautiful baby girl, Esther, was born on March 24, 2017. I am so blessed to have her. I stayed at the hospital for four days. When I was ready to be released, I asked my mom if I could stay with her for a short time until I could find someone who would allow me and the baby to stay with them. I had to stay in Canada until I could get a birth certificate for Esther. Then I would be able to go home to Niagara Falls, New York.

The next day after going to my mom's house, she kicked me and the baby out because the baby cried all night. I cried, was scared, and was suffering much.

I called Brian in Niagara Falls. I told him he needed to pick up Esther and me. He drove four hours to get us and take us to a hotel. We stayed at the hotel until I was able to get Esther's birth certificate.

I realized I only had Brian. No one else cared about me or the baby. No one was willing to help me. I didn't have friends in Canada. I hated the Canadian system for not helping me. I hated my family. There was no mercy.

Brian and I lived in Niagara Falls, New York, for a year and a half. I found out in January I was pregnant with Mesha. He was born September 5, 2018, in Flower Mound, Texas. He was a very special baby.

I dreamed about Mesha a lot. I saw him as a grown boy in my dream. He was so happy and smart. In my last dream of him, I saw him graduate from high school. Mesha said to me in the dream, "Thank you, my beautiful Mama," and he hugged me. I smiled and cried at the same time.

When Mesha was born, I thought he looked like my brother, Daniel. Why would it have to be Daniel that he reminded me of? I dreamed GOOD about Mesha; now, I only saw bad about him because he reminded me of DANIEL! Why did I have to constantly be reminded of Daniel?

Mesha had jaundice. He had yellow skin and yellow eyes. The hospital wouldn't help me when I told them I needed a blue light. They wouldn't give it to me because I was deaf and they didn't believe I needed it. It seemed that hearing people were so privileged, getting help, but I didn't! Mesha suffered with jaundice for two months, and I suffered with postpartum depression.

*****

On Sunday, February 3, 2019, we were at Allie's house in Garland, Texas, to watch football on TV and to socialize. Allie was a friend of mine from our church. Most of the children were playing upstairs. My daughter, Esther, who was only 23 months old, was sitting on the couch, watching kids' songs on YouTube. My son, Mesha, five months old, was sleeping.

I was sitting on the couch, as well, thinking about finding freedom from my past. I knew I needed to let go and to forgive those who hurt me. I looked at Mesha and struggled inside of myself. I believed he looked so much like my brother, Daniel, so Mesha's face was a constant reminder of the abuse I suffered from Daniel.

I turned to Kameron, another friend from our church, who was sitting behind me. I said, "I am ready." Kameron knew I carried a heavy energy of hate and anger inside of me. He knew I needed help, love, and support to go on. I hadn't told Kameron, but Kameron knew my HEART, and God had called him to help me let go of my past.

Kameron called Kendrick to get ready. My husband, Brian, and our other friends from church,

Mark, Kenecia, Daniel, and Allie, all encouraged me to hit pillows to forget my past. First, I went to Allie's bedroom to change out of my dress into shorts and a T-shirt. When I came out of the bedroom, I saw myself as a spirit standing in front of me. I looked like I was about eight years old. After I looked at it for a minute, it was gone.

I walked to the living room. As he held my shoulder, Kendrick prayed that I would let go of my past and release those who hurt me. I could see what looked like smoke behind him as he prayed. He felt goosebumps, and his heart burned. The others joined him praying for me, and their prayers were powerful.

I had been carrying my past for years and years. I started hitting the pillows, screaming and explaining why I held onto my hatred and anger for so long. I continued to hit the pillows. Kendrick touched my forehead, and I fell down, feeling so much lighter; the heavy weight of anger and hate was gone. I looked at my son and noticed he didn't look like my brother, Daniel, any longer.

I was free.

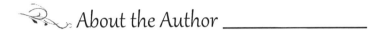 ## About the Author

Jennifer A. Hertneky, 26 years old, is deaf. She lives with her deaf husband, Brian, and their two beautiful children in Frisco, Texas. Born in Toronto, Ontario, Canada, she was raised in Brampton, Ontario. She graduated from George Brown College in Toronto and earned a certificate as a Makeup Artist. In July, 2014, she was a contestant as Miss Canada at the Miss and Mister Deaf International, Inc., held in England. She has the gifts/spirit of a Christian. She enjoys having the freedom of being a stay-at-home mom to Esther and Mesha while running her pet sitting business from her home.

To connect with Jennifer:

You can email her at
jennifer.matti@gmail.com.

Made in the USA
Lexington, KY
26 November 2019